LAST DIET BOOK

(You'll Ever Need!)

by
DR. DAVID FISCH

CCC PUBLICATIONS

Published by

CCC Publications
9725 Lurline Avenue
Chatsworth, CA 91311

Manufactured in the United States of America

Cover © 1997 CCC Publications

Cover/Interior production by Oasis Graphics

ISBN: 1-57644-055-9

If your local U.S. bookstore is out of stock, copies of this
book may be obtained by mailing check or money order
for $4.99 per book (plus $2.50 to cover postage and
handling) to: CCC Publications, 9725 Lurline Avenue;
Chatsworth, CA 91311.

Pre-publication Edition - 6/97

EAT
LESS!

EAT LESS!

EAT LESS!

EAT
LESS!

EAT LESS!

EAT

LESS!

EAT LESS!

EAT LESS!

EAT LESS!

EAT
LESS!

EAT
LESS!

EAT

LESS!

EAT LESS!

EAT LESS!

EAT LESS!

EAT

LESS!

EAT LESS!

EAT

LESS!

EAT LESS!

EAT LESS!

EAT LESS!

EAT

LESS!

EAT LESS!

EAT LESS!

EAT LESS!

EAT LESS!

EAT
LESS!

EAT

LESS!

EAT LESS!

EAT LESS!

EAT

LESS!

EAT

LESS!

EAT

LESS!

EAT LESS!

EAT

LESS!

EAT LESS!

EAT LESS!

EAT LESS!

EAT LESS!

EAT LESS!

EAT LESS!

EAT
LESS!

EAT

LESS!

EAT LESS!

EAT

LESS!

EAT

LESS!

EAT LESS!

EAT LESS!

EAT

LESS!

EAT

LESS!

EAT

LESS!

EAT LESS!

EAT LESS!

EAT

LESS!

EAT LESS!

EAT LESS!

EAT
LESS!

EAT LESS!

EAT

LESS!

EAT

LESS!

EAT
LESS!

EAT

LESS!

EAT
LESS!

EAT

LESS!

EAT LESS!

EAT

LESS!

EAT LESS!

EAT
LESS!

EAT LESS!

EAT

LESS!

EAT

LESS!

EAT LESS!

EAT LESS!

EAT

LESS!

EAT LESS!

EAT

LESS!

EAT LESS!

EAT LESS!

EAT LESS!

EAT LESS!

EAT

LESS!

EAT LESS!

EAT LESS!

EAT LESS!

EAT LESS!

EAT

LESS!

EAT LESS!

EAT LESS!

EAT
LESS!

EAT

LESS!

EAT LESS!

EAT
LESS!

EAT
LESS!

TITLES BY CCC PUBLICATIONS

Blank Books ($3.99)
SEX AFTER BABY
SEX AFTER 30
SEX AFTER 40
SEX AFTER 50

Retail $4.95 – $4.99
30 – DEAL WITH IT!
40 – DEAL WITH IT!
50 – DEAL WITH IT!
60 – DEAL WITH IT!
RETIRED – DEAL WITH IT!
"?" book
POSITIVELY PREGNANT
CAN SEX IMPROVE YOUR GOLF?
THE COMPLETE BOOGER BOOK
FLYING FUNNIES
MARITAL BLISS & OXYMORONS
THE VERY VERY SEXY ADULT DOT-TO-DOT BOOK
THE DEFINITIVE FART BOOK
THE COMPLETE WIMP'S GUIDE TO SEX
THE CAT OWNER'S SHAPE UP MANUAL
THE OFFICE FROM HELL
FITNESS FANATICS
YOUNGER MEN ARE BETTER THAN RETIN-A
BUT OSSIFER, IT'S NOT MY FAULT
YOU KNOW YOU'RE AN OLD FART WHEN...
1001 WAYS TO PROCRASTINATE
HORMONES FROM HELL II
SHARING THE ROAD WITH IDIOTS
THE GREATEST ANSWERING MACHINE MESSAGES
WHAT DO WE DO NOW??
HOW TO TALK YOU WAY OUT OF A TRAFFIC TICKET
THE BOTTOM HALF
LIFE'S MOST EMBARRASSING MOMENTS
HOW TO ENTERTAIN PEOPLE YOU HATE
YOUR GUIDE TO CORPORATE SURVIVAL
THE SUPERIOR PERSON'S GUIDE
GIFTING RIGHT
NO HANG-UPS (Volumes I, II & III – $3.95 ea.)
TOTALLY OUTRAGEOUS BUMPER-SNICKERS ($2.95)

Retail $5.95
SINGLE WOMEN VS. MARRIED WOMEN
TAKE A WOMAN'S WORD FOR IT
SEXY CROTCHWORD PUZZLES
SO, YOU'RE GETTING MARRIED
YOU KNOW HE'S A WOMANIZING SLIMEBALL WHEN...
GETTING OLD SUCKS
WHY GOD MAKES BALD GUYS
OH BABY!
PMS CRAZED: TOUCH ME AND I'LL KILL YOU!

OVER THE HILL – DEAL WITH IT!
WHY MEN ARE CLUELESS
THE BOOK OF WHITE TRASH
THE ART OF MOONING
GOLFAHOLICS
CRINKLED 'N' WRINKLED
SMART COMEBACKS FOR STUPID QUESTIONS
YIKES! IT'S ANOTHER BIRTHDAY
SEX IS A GAME
SEX AND YOUR STARS
SIGNS YOUR SEX LIFE IS DEAD
40 AND HOLDING YOUR OWN
50 AND HOLDING YOUR OWN
MALE BASHING: WOMEN'S FAVORITE PASTIME
THINGS YOU CAN DO WITH A USELESS MAN
MORE THINGS YOU CAN DO WITH A USELESS MAN
THE WORLD'S GREATEST PUT-DOWN LINES
LITTLE INSTRUCTION BOOK OF THE RICH & FAMOUS
WELCOME TO YOUR MIDLIFE CRISIS
GETTING EVEN WITH THE ANSWERING MACHINE
ARE YOU A SPORTS NUT?
MEN ARE PIGS / WOMEN ARE BITCHES
THE BETTER HALF
ARE WE DYSFUNCTIONAL YET?
TECHNOLOGY BYTES!
50 WAYS TO HUSTLE YOUR FRIENDS
HORMONES FROM HELL
HUSBANDS FROM HELL
KILLER BRAS & Other Hazards Of The 50's
IT'S BETTER TO BE OVER THE HILL THAN UNDER IT
HOW TO REALLY PARTY!!!
WORK SUCKS!
THE PEOPLE WATCHER'S FIELD GUIDE
THE ABSOLUTE LAST CHANCE DIET BOOK
FOR MEN ONLY (How To Survive Marriage)
THE UGLY TRUTH ABOUT MEN
NEVER A DULL CARD
THE LITTLE BOOK OF ROMANTIC LIES
THE LITTLE BOOK OF CORPORATE LIES ($6.95)
RED HOT MONOGAMY ($6.95)
LOVE DAT CAT ($6.95)
HOW TO SURVIVE A JEWISH MOTHER ($6.95)
WHY MEN DON'T HAVE A CLUE ($7.99)
LADIES, START YOUR ENGINES! ($7.99)

NO HANG-UPS – CASSETTES Retail $5.98

Vol. I:	GENERAL MESSAGES (M or F)
Vol. II:	BUSINESS MESSAGES (M or F)
Vol. III:	'R' RATED MESSAGES (M or F)
Vol. V:	CELEBRI-TEASE